The Miracle On Overseas Highway

THE MIRACLE ON OVERSEAS HIGHWAY

God's Saving Grace

KAROL SUSAN HARRELSON

XULON PRESS

Xulon Press
2301 Lucien Way #415
Maitland, FL 32751
407.339.4217
www.xulonpress.com

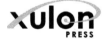

© 2022 by Karol Susan Harrelson

Contribution by: Lynn Grafton

All rights reserved solely by the author. The author guarantees all contents are original and do not infringe upon the legal rights of any other person or work. No part of this book may be reproduced in any form without the permission of the author.

Due to the changing nature of the Internet, if there are any web addresses, links, or URLs included in this manuscript, these may have been altered and may no longer be accessible. The views and opinions shared in this book belong solely to the author and do not necessarily reflect those of the publisher. The publisher therefore disclaims responsibility for the views or opinions expressed within the work.

Unless otherwise indicated, Scripture quotations taken from the New King James Version (NKJV). Copyright © 1982 by Thomas Nelson, Inc. Used by permission. All rights reserved.

Paperback ISBN-13: 978-1-66286-187-1
Ebook ISBN-13: 978-1-66286-188-8

Preface

There is nothing special about me, it is He Who lives in me.

Galatian's 2:20
"I have been crucified with Christ; it is no longer I who live, but Christ lives in me; and the life which now live in the flesh, I live by faith in the Son of God, who loved me and gave Himself for me."

These are my life verses:

Proverbs 3:5&6
5 "Trust in the Lord with all your heart and lean not on your own understanding. 6 In all your ways acknowledge Him and He shall direct your paths."
These verses are so special to me. They have seen me through very dark times in my life. They speak to me in ways that I know without a doubt, He is carrying me, and He will always be carrying me. I have had troubling times in my life, but what I am about to tell you, is by far the darkest and most painful time I, and my family have ever experienced.

I am a miracle of God. He has saved my life so many times. Times when I should not have been doing what I was doing, and this the most terrifying time, the car accident that changed my, and my family's life forever. He has been faithful to me repeatedly; He will always remain faithful to me and those who believe. He will keep you whole, He loves us, we are His children. He has nothing but love for His children

My immediate family is my husband Terry of thirty years, thirty-two together, Terry Jr. (Christine) my grandchildren, Ty, Macey, Glade and Colt and Tammy (Chuck) and my grandchildren Lizzy, Damien, Nola and Cora, from Terry's first marriage, Sarah, and her new husband Patrick. I come from a family of five; Bill the oldest, Mary or Honey, who passed away in twenty eighteen, Lynn, and my baby brother Karl, Karl and I are fifteen-months apart. My husband Terry and Karl are the best of friends.

I am a registered nurse, one Monday as I was traveling to school to become an ICU nurse, a big box truck ran the red light at the entrance to my neighborhood in the Florida Keys, I was in the wrong place at the wrong time.

He hit me pushing me into a light pole and destroying a bench, thank God no one was there at the time. I went into a coma at once; I suffer from a traumatic brain injury. There are times in a group of people, the noise overwhelms me, I become easily distracted. Headaches come easily. Confusion comes often. Your brain controls everything about you. My husband Terry was first on the scene. How horrible he must have felt. I was running late that day to the Academy. I never made it. I spent the next five months in five different hospitals.

My brain injury is at the brain stem, all the centers for breathing, speech, and so forth. I was intubated. My heart stopped twice, once in the helicopter, once at Jackson Memorial hospital, all from trauma. From what my husband tells me, I was given two injections to wake me, they did not work. My powerful God woke me.

So, you see I truly am His miracle, people do not survive major accidents like mine. The only reason I am here drafting this book is because of His grace and loving kindness.

At the hospital I worked for; I worked as a floor nurse, Palliative Care nurse, and once a month, chairing a cancer support group, working for a local nursing agency with regular patients, weekly.

Just what used to be simple to me, typing, cursive writing, driving a car, getting myself dressed for the day, all my daily activities, everything we take for granted. This is all so much harder now, but I know that Jesus is with me every moment. In the blink of an eye, the tables were turned, I was the patient.

Your life can change in instant; I was an incredibly careful driver. That morning, I had the red light at the entrance to my neighborhood. I looked both ways before I started to cross, I never saw this big box truck, he came extremely fast running the red light, hitting me on the passenger side, pushing me into a light pole, destroying a pedestrian bench; and his truck ended up in the woods.

When I awoke from the coma after 3 months, I had absolutely no idea what had happened to me... I must have been in ICU. I had one nurse, there was cloudiness around her face. It was dreamlike. I was so thirsty from being intubated for three months. The most important part of bedside nursing.

Joshua 1:9
Be strong and of good courage; do not be afraid or dismayed, for the Lord your God is with you wherever you go

Karol Susan Harrelson

There are so many times I think about that day. Especially when we live in the same town where it happened. I am trying to be strong. I often find myself in prayer, that God will keep me safe throughout the day, that I say the right things to people, or I just carry on a conversation with Him. He always listens to me.

I come from strong women, My Mother Mary Frances was a registered nurse, and later in life became an ARNP. I had a sister, Mary who passed in 2018 who worked for a physician at one time and was in nursing school.

My sister, Lynn whom I am remarkably close with became a registered nurse. After she graduated high school, she married her high school sweetheart, had three girls who are like my girls, to this day. I am so enormously proud of each of them. They are all beautiful women, strong, resilient, and forgiving, just as Jesus tells us to be.

My family, the women were all nurses. My maternal great grandmother was a nurse and lived to be one hundred. My maternal grandmother rode the Flagler Railway down to Key West in the thirties to volunteer after the thirty-five hurricanes. My mother, Mary Frances was a registered nurse who became a nurse practitioner. She was in the first graduating class of nurse practitioners at the University of Miami in the seventies. That tells you how long my family has been in Homestead.

My Father, Karl, was a lieutenant on the police force in Homestead, Florida where I was born and raised. My paternal grandmother Eunice, cooked for the hospital in Homestead, Redland School, and South Dade High School. My family has always been in service to others. Service to others, is a very noble action. Jesus was always giving to others.

I have many friends who are nurses, they are all incredibly special to me. I still have contact with so many of them. Jacqueline who I have known since my daughter was in middle school, Mary, who I still get together with Sharon who trained me as a clinical partner when I first began in the nursing field, Beverley who precepted me as a clinical partner, Therese who precepted me as a nurse, and many more. They all taught me with love and direction. There are far too many to mention, but they are all very important to me, and I love and respect them all.

When I awoke from the coma after 3 months, I had absolutely no idea what had happened to me... I must have been in ICU. I had one nurse, there was cloudiness around her face. It was dreamlike. I was so thirsty from intubation for three months. She could only give me glycerin sticks, unaware of how I could swallow. The most important part of bedside nursing is keeping the patient safe. I had a feeding tube, Terry told me I pulled it out, and had to have it put back in, I had no idea where I was, what happened to me, nothing.

Terry had no idea I had woken up, he walked in find me awake, he called everyone. Then the hard part started. Recovery and therapy. Recovery is hard, I am still recovering after seven years. A nurse practitioner told me once my disabilities may be lifelong. I was so active before. It is very frustrating to be so limited. My speech is much better at first in just babbled, my daughter Sarah, told me to over enunciate my words, which makes a huge difference.

I pride myself on being intelligent. I am very caring and loyal; I would go beyond for those in need. I am an excellent nurse I still hold my license, but I do not practice anymore. I just know for me; I cannot go one single moment without Jesus. He is the Master of my life. My way maker, my Prince of peace. My everything. I do not know how people can go through life on their own. He gives me strength and purpose.

I hope this book will inspire someone, change someone's life for the better. I do know when you talk to Christ He listens. He is your friend, Father, and Helper. He is our way maker.

Seven years may seem like a long time, but, then again, everything is relative, and an experience, even a single moment can bring changes in our lives such as we could have never imagined. As soon as Karol was able to begin her life again, that is, breathing on her own, walking, talking and managing everything we take for granted, I remember she stayed focused on what could it be that God wanted from her now.

Karol and Terry had about finished raising Sarah Frances who was in her second year of college in West Palm Beach. It had just been a few years since Karol had conducted what she thought was God's plan for her and certainly a significant life goal. Though she had her family and work and school, Karol spent much of her time at our mother's side during the final years before Momma lost her battle with lung cancer. This was the most awkward thing that anyone in our family had ever experienced. There are just no words to describe the deep gripping void when you have to say good-by to your mother, forever. As wonderful as the knowledge is you'll see your loved one again in heaven someday, nothing could console us then. That was Momma. Our mother, Mary Frances was a Registered Nurse, in fact she was also in the first graduating class of Nurse Practitioners in the State of Florida. She was the center of our family, our anchor. Describing her would require another book, so I'll just say she was and always be profoundly loved and respected. My point, Karol also is a registered nurse, as am I and my daughter, Mary Ann. You could say it runs in the family as our great-grandmother, Lillian Atkins was a nurse in the late 1800's in Lewes Delaware. I'm certain Karol's relationship with our mother and experiencing the struggle with her had a considerable influence on her decision to become a nurse. But too, my sister already had all the makings of an amazing RN as I hope she'll share with you some of her passion and accomplishments during her far too brief career, cut short by a single moment in time. This book is just the beginning of Karol's calling and I'm so proud of my sister, who always, always" Loves you more!"

Homestead was a wonderful place to be coming up in the 50's and 60's. I was born in the summer of 1949, the last of Momma's three children with, Ed Pacetti who also lost his life to cancer at such an early age of 32. I was only 3, Bill 9 and Honey 6. Actually, Honey got her nickname from our father, who was so taken by his first baby girls' beautiful golden hair. Honey's name was Mary Montese, after our mother and her best friend, my father's sister. We lost Honey unexpectedly three years ago and still the void is as palatable as if it happened yesterday. Through our childhood she was a few steps ahead of me, leading me, showing me, advising me, you know, the things big sisters do. Honey was my idol. Many times, since that early November Monday morning, Karol has listened quietly and responded with just the right words to console, support and encourage me through our loss. You see, the youngest of us three girls, turns out, Karol has an amazing ability to recognize and sort out troubling emotions like sadness, anxiety or grief, and place everything into perspective in a more hopeful, healing way. And now, after all these years, my little sister Karol is my rock.

I remember as if it were yesterday, standing in Aunt Mosely's living room the day Momma married my stepfather, Karl Greer. I was seven and so excited to be a part of the excitement. There's a very cherished family picture of everyone standing together under an archway, both sets of parents at their sides, my deeply loved grandmother, Beatrice Arthur and Grandfather Skipper and my new grandparents, Granny and Grandaddy Greer. I sensed the joy after the years following my father's death in which Momma probably just managed to survive.

Then came the fun years of my childhood, thanks to our grandmother Bea, Karol and I agree we were both raised by her. Following our grandfather's death Bea moved to our house and that was probably the single best thing that ever happened in my life. Bea still had her house on Biscayne and if I asked Momma once I asked her a thousand times, "Can I spend the night with Bea?". Karol and I have the same wonderful memories only from different years because Bea, was always there for both of us and there's much more to this special relationship including summers in the mountains of North Carolina or at the beach in Delaware, school shopping, Bayfront Park, Dairy Queen. She even drove us each year to Miami to watch the orange Bowl parade and a really special occasion was the Snow-White ice-cream dessert at Burdines, way up overlooking the skyline. All of it, the two of us were given the best "jump start" on life thru our experiences with our mother's mother Beatrice Arthur. This, of course takes nothing from Momma, as both Karol and I will tell you in a heartbeat that Mary Frances Greer was, is and will always be the strongest and most respected person in our lives, not to mention most accomplished and a perfect example to which anyone could follow.

So, in 1956 our new family of five is coming along, with Bea, of course right there in the mix to get the kids where they need to go, get Anna, our housekeeper, who we loved, back and forth. I remember there was a lot going on. About the time I started helping Bea with the dishes every evening after supper, seems like it was always just the two of us as Bill and Honey, now ten and thirteen, always had something else they had to do, Though Momma was incredibly good at accomplishing so many things and all at once it seemed like, she must have been challenged many times. Though I didn't think of it then, considering it now, it took a talented woman to manage successfully all of her projects of which she had many, not just a full-time job but a developing career that not only diversified from clinical to industrial nursing with Aerojet but eventually included a higher education and a practice at Community Health Incorporated. Did I mention her Merle Norman Studio or buying and selling antique furniture or marketing jewelry or the City Council or even the Key she was given to Date County. Karol and I are not kidding when we say we had a remarkable mother, one in a line of strong women.

The wonderful years in Homestead were just beginning for me. But back to the kitchen thing for a bit. One of the really nice things about our family now was that my new dad liked to cook. His Police Department schedule often allowed him the time fix supper which helped Momma who at one point was coming home in the afternoon when she managed a physician's office or when she had to sleep before the drive to Baptist Hospital in Kendall for night shift Labor and Delivery. Karl Greer's fried chicken was the best. He once told me his secret was to salt and pepper the flour, also hot with the lid on. So now, Karol's fried chicken is the best, mine, not so much.

I now had extra special birthdays which was July 5th. For a kid at this age birthdays are a big deal and the excitement for me doubled. My stepdad played softball on the Police Department team. He was the catcher and I remember sitting in the bleachers with Momma and Bea almost directly behind him. That was fun enough but then when it was the fourth of July game and fireworks afterwards, then my birthday the next day. Boy that was the best. As Honey once told me we really did have a good childhood. Momma saw to that. Little did I know, we were about to grow as a family, and I cannot describe my excitement over the news of a baby coming. It must have been a profound thought for me to see my mother pregnant as I remember very vividly the image of her in her powder blue robe, pregnant with a baby! She seemed so capable of anything, and the blessing was repeated again in two years when my youngest brother, Karl was born. Life was the best is had ever been. I soon had another sister and brother and this time in my life was a big reason of why I write coming up in Homestead during those years was wonderful. God was so good to us and though eventually as we grew older and experienced life's disappointments and heartaches, the foundations were being laid so well that we were given all we needed and more to weather any storm.

Another thing I remember very well, though I hadn't had reason to consider this for so many years. I was invited into a conversation that was taking place with Momma my new dad and I'm pretty sure at least Bea was there. Though our grandmother had her own life with church and bridge friends as well as still spending summers in Delaware with our great-grandmother, she always seemed to be with us as well, and especially on every important occasion. Looking back, Bea and Momma must have had an understanding. or perhaps It was just on her own that she became a constant presence when we lost my father. This life changing event, my sister Karol and I both agree had a wonderfully positive impact on both of us. Looking back, we were so fortunate Bea was there to help raise us up because we now share a common understanding of many important things in life as faith, family and our love of God and our savior Jesus Christ. Oh, and back to me, at nine years old and about to get a new baby sister. It's true that I was asked, and I certainly did interject my opinion about her name. Karol Susan was finalized when I agreed I liked that as I had a Carol Sue in my dance class, and I liked my sister's name even better.

Karol coming along when she did have a big influence in my life, both when she arrived and as the years passed through each phase of our lives, my sister has always, always been right there for me. Her birth and then watching her grow from a baby to my little sister, the cutest, sweetest thing you ever saw. When I was only maybe twelve, I started my own baby-sitting business in Momma's living room. We once had a little "Tea Party". The all-girl toddlers were dressed up, in their crinoline skirts, Karol included. Though she was in the group, she was also my little sister and that just gave me the confidence in my first, new baby-sitting "business". We had so much fun that day.

I hope to find a picture that was taken that day. It will absolutely show the pure innocent joy of life from those years. And maybe or maybe not, considering publishing constraints, I can share another picture, as incidental as it might seem, of a two-year-old with golden locks, standing on a coffee table in front of Momma's fireplace, in an "itsy-bitsy-tiny-winy, yellow-polka dot bikini. So cute, so precious, best yet I set her up there and took that picture. My, my little sister.

We each had our different lives going on. Quickly I moved into my teens and found love, better put, fell deeply in love at only fifteen. Nine and a half years age difference may seem like enough to separate interest and activities for even sisters, but that never seemed to happen. I always felt a special connection to my younger sister, even with my three-year older sister, Honey whom I shared our bedroom with. We had the southeast corner of the house, windows on three sides with tropical breezed always coming through. We shared those amazing, magical years together in our white French Provincial bedroom that became a place to hold many hopes and dreams, secrets and disappointments and a sisters love and support even to this day.

Soon I would be a mom, and this is the time I began to see the qualities in Karol that would carry through with her as she followed me into adulthood. At just ten, now remember, right about the time I began babysitting, Karol would call and say," Do you need a baby-sitter today?" She genuinely adored my three girls, Heather, Mary Ann and Brooke and they loved her too. We have so many good memories from those years and not once was Karol not willing and available to spend time with us. I'm smiling at this moment when I think of the occasion of another picture taken of Karol pushing the girls in a stroller at Crandon Park Zoo. Years later after we moved to Georgia, I came home to attend Karol's baby shower. There was a good-sized crowd with a lot of Momma's friends there. I was visiting with those I hadn't seen in a long time and there was a lot of noise with ladies visiting and celebrating the occasion. Suddenly there was quiet. I looked to see Karol standing, very pregnant, holding the picture of her and my girls from Crandon Park Zoo in front on her, tears falling. That day will never fade from either of our memories.

As the years passed by, Karol in Florida, now a mom too, and me in Georgia with two more, boys this time, Ben, and Aaron, we did lose touch. Looking back, I can hardly see how that was possible, but life has a way of pulling you from even the most valued people in our life. Time just happened but nothing happened or ever will to the respect, love and adoration I have for my sister Karol. I've shared memories, experiences, things that occurred to influence both of as we've grown and more importantly how we've reacted and conducted ourselves as we became adults. Our primary educations were different. I graduated from South Dade High School and Karol from Colonial Christian. Both of us returned after marriage and children for our RN degrees. Karol 's never been far from her faith, her beliefs, and her church. She worked as a church secretary before going after her long-coveted goal of becoming a nurse.

This is where my sister's experiences culminate with the amazing person that she is, and I personally know, she always has been. When she was just a little thing, she was always smiling. As a child she would show a genuine concern for the welfare of others, always wanting to make things better, especially when she recognized a need. It was never about her and she'd look for ways to help in everything. The long, drawn-out years of our mother's battle with cancer, were followed in no time with her dad's struggle before losing him as well. During this time there were many opportunities for learning about what many make a concerted effort to avoid, and that is caring for and more importantly comforting someone who's dying. That is, someone you love very deeply, someone who's meant so much to you, and in this case, both mother and father. I believe God was preparing Karol.

I wasn't surprised at my sister's decision to pursue a nursing career about the time Sarah Frances was in high school. I remember my mix of emotions in hearing her excitement over each accomplishment during that time. She excelled academically, again no surprise, and with every call I shared her joy but with it came a linger of sadness when we'd both take pause to express our confidence that Momma was so proud of her too, but from heaven. There's just no getting around that desire of a mother's acceptance, anytime, anywhere. So, for that, I felt bad for my sister, but God was working, and we grew even closer.

The transition from nursing student to RN in the clinical setting is challenge enough, but Karol had her sites set still on her heart's desire. This time it was to finally reach for what it was she felt God was preparing her for. She pursued credentialing in providing care during the end of life. In my own career I had never personally known another nurse who had chosen that career path. Once again, no surprise here, but with a profoundly deep admiration, I loved my sister even more. She didn't get done after all that time and heartache. Instead, Karol took her experiences, added her education and was now refining her skills to answer what she felt strongly was her calling.

Everything had finally fallen into place. Sarah Frances was in college now, Karol was well settled in and enjoying her work and new nursing colleagues and friends at Mariners Hospital. Besides the classes she had already taken for Hospice training (a part of the plan to enhance this service at Mariner's) Karol was currently taking a Trauma course. In fact, she had a clinical scheduled at Rider Trauma Center in Miami the morning everything changed for her, Terry, Sarah Frances, our entire family, and the Florida Keys medical community.

Karol Susan Harrelson

July 6, 2015, will forever linger in our thoughts. Like my memory of sitting in my band classroom in the 7th grade the day Kennedy was shot or 9/11, we mention this very morning from time to time. I have thought about our phone call many times, but for Terry I can't imagine the nightmare for him that morning. Karol had just left the house and was only as far as a few blocks away, close enough for him to hear the impact. The rest doesn't matter. That there was delay for the Jaws of Life, that Karol arrested twice, that someone from another country, driving a box truck didn't stop for a red light and Karol was propelled before her car wrapped around a utility pole. What does matter now is that she survived the flight to Rider that morning, not the student from her group but as the patient. It's just plain gripping still to even think about that day seven years later and the first days in the trauma center, then the early weeks at Kendall that turned into months where Karol lay sleeping.

It took six days to arrange for the five of us to leave work a make the trip to Coral Gables where Karol remained in the trauma center, still unstable and a large effort happening to save her life, which didn't look hopeful. July 6th was a Friday. We were at my sister's bedside the following Friday at 3:00 in the afternoon after driving thru the night from Georgia. There was no mention of question or hesitation, all my children were going with me, except for Heather in Texas who stayed in constant communication. The urgency was like weight. I remember the daily, sometimes hourly calls and when the phone rang, my heart would drop. Please God don't take Karol and especially not before we can get to her.

Terry was amazing. I saw the anguish in his eyes, but he was smiling when he greeted us. When I listened to his updates he spoke ever so calmly and never once broke into any outward emotion when I knew he had to be afraid for what the next hour would bring. I could literally feel his adoration. As he explained what we were seeing, he would take pause, look to Karol's face and smile, then go back to explaining. This observation was not my imagination. I knew Karol and Terry had a good marriage and they had a church family. I thought I pretty much knew my brother-in-law of twenty-three years. Over the next three days I saw the Terry I had not known before. He never expresses outwardly any of the anguish he had to have been feeling inside. Their whole life had been turned upside down. Karol had graduated a couple of years earlier which meant an RN's income. But I'm sure that thought was the furthest thing from Terry's mind. Still, the financial aspect and certainly that all of the hard work and sacrifice, had just been completely wiped out, Karol's dreams shattered in one moment in time, and not at all by her doing. Terry stayed so calm and cautiously positive. Considering what he was up against there was only one reason for his composure, which is faith. His wife was covered everywhere with tubing and equipment, the noise of machines running, and alarms was constant, and you had to speak up to talk over it all. Ryder Trauma Center is one very large circular room with at least a dozen beds all the way around the wall. The beds were full, and every patient was acutely critical. It was overwhelming just to be in the room.

We came right to the trauma enter, my four adult children and I couldn't get to Karol's bedside fast enough. We knew the situation, but we had to see her for ourselves before it could actually be real, if that makes any sense. Nothing could have prepared me for this, and I remember thinking Karol comes from a line of strong women, this will take every bit of fight she has in her. I was so afraid for her and even more afraid for myself if this also makes any sense. You see, I know my sister's faith was strong. Without a doubt I knew she had a personal relationship with our Lord and Savior Jesus Christ, and she believed completely in God, our heavenly father's love and his grace and his mercy. Karol was saved and I had no concerns about her having any fear for her future. She wouldn't want to leave Terry and Sarah, but I knew Karol trusted God in everything and would yield to his will. But I was so not ready to give my sister up, not now, not this way. Over the next three days, my prayers were desperate bouts of pleading, begging God to let her stay with us. But honestly that Friday afternoon, one week into this ordeal, it wasn't looking too good. She had been to surgery for a fractured leg and arm, her spleen had been removed during an exploratory lap for hemorrhaging. There were more procedures to relieve the increased pressure from her brain injury. All the while Karol lay sleeping. She didn't appear to be perceiving pain which was concerning to me. But the cold hard fact was, my little sister laid there completely still, as is she were sleeping peacefully but she was in a coma, and I was in a nightmare. Please dear Lord let her live.

We had to gown, mask and glove before going in. There were no restrictions in visitors. I figured because for many of the families it would be the last few minutes with their loved one. Ben surprised me. It was just more than he felt he could do to go in and see his Aunt Karol like that. Aaron surprised me even more. He didn't slow down after he suited up. He went directly to Karol's bedside and studied everything he saw, almost as if he was taking a survey. That warmed my heart so to see the genuine love and concern. Aaron wanted to know the extent of Karol's injuries, maybe so he could judge for himself if he thought she could survive this or so he could have a list in his thoughts when he petitioned God in his prayers. Mary Ann my ICU nurse immediately engaged the staff for answers to her questions. Brooke and I just stood beside Karol, touching her, wishing we could hold her and make everything all right, but we could not. It was beyond our control and only God knew his plan and what was in the future for my sister if anything at all.

It was getting to be early evening when we arrived at the Colonnade in Coral Gables. It worked out that I had found nice accommodations, two rooms, a roof-top pool overlooking the skyline. The Colonnade was beautiful, lots of pink marble, perfect for events and an impressive history explained in pictures lining the grand hallways. It had a Morton's, all that one could ask for on a vacation, and for a second that's what it seemed like we were doing, but then reality would hit like a ton of bricks. The kids and I enjoyed one another's company as it had been a long time since we had been on vacations together. We had a wonderful dinner out, all on Aaron. I suppose it was a nice distraction for the time we were there but not with Karol. Late the Friday of our arrival, a week after the accident Karol was transferred to Kindred, a long-term intensive care facility within a couple of blocks of where we were staying. So, we managed to make the best of an unplanned trip from north Georgia to south Florida. All the last-minute arranging went smoothly from everyone getting unscheduled leave from work to consensus in the group of five on everything we did for five days. What a road trip. Except for one thing, our Karol lie sleeping while we were trying to behave as if there wasn't complete devastation hanging over us. There was lots of talk about every detail concerning Karol. We were all struck by the fact that, despite what everything surrounding her actually meant, she looked at peace, literally as if she was just asleep.

We visited Karol every day, every opportunity given to us. Sometimes we took turns, sometimes together. Countless people from literally, around the world were praying for

Karol, Terry and Sarah Frances. I felt especially good about that as we know scripture tells us that if two or more come together... I just knew God had to be holding my sister in his arms somehow, protecting her from all that her body was going thru. I never saw expressions of pain or fear or anxiety. And I know Karol well, if she had been able, she would have been worrying herself to no end over how this was affecting Terry and Sarah. I was grateful then when I felt a sense she was being sheltered. And I'll be eternally grateful all of my days for all of the love and support as well as the countless prayers on Karol's behalf. God was listening and boy did he answer.

Three long month's later when we heard the amazing, wonderful news that Karol was awake, well there are just no words. My own joy was mixed with a lot of concern for what lie ahead. How much of Karol had we gotten back? The arm and leg injuries I knew, at least would impact her mobility. That part was workable. I knew my sister would give 110% of what was asked of her regarding physical therapy. There hadn't been recent updates on the initial concerns about internal organ damage so that I didn't have a clue about. Then there was the biggest insult of all, the injuries to Karol's brain. They were not from blunt force trauma, rather she had defused, "multi-focal" damage, sort of like "shaken baby syndrome". The impact to her van catapulted her during which time she was thrown around thus shaking her brain within the skull. These types of injuries are about impossible to predict a prognosis and you can imagine back then, this was what was foremost in our thoughts. Would Karol return to us as the warm, loving, deeply caring person we knew, so smart and already accomplished in her career or had her hopes and dreams for the future been taken away.

The days had turned into weeks, then weeks to months. I remember thinking so many times, she's still alive. Hope remained ever present though now fall was coming and Karol was still sleeping. No one could answer the questions, is this all there is, is this God's will? I'm pretty sure the entire group of a large prayerful community was not accepting that notion. I know I couldn't. And so, we kept on waiting and praying, never to give up hope. Terry kept his routine going, day in and day out. It was probably better Sarah was at West Palm because his load was about impossible. It's no quick trip between Key Largo and Coral Gables but Terry traveled north to see Karol after laying sheet rock all day every day. I can't see how this wouldn't take its toll. But then again, his faith was his drive, and his Karol was waiting, unaware, protected while her brain needed this time to heal. And then one day, that moment of God's choosing Karol was awake, waiting for her faithful, devoted husband. I cannot imagine the joy and profound appreciation for what so many had been asking for three long months.

In Georgia we were elated to put it mildly. Immediately I went into a repeat mode from July. This time Mary Ann and I were on the road within twenty-four hours. The dark months of struggling to keep hoping God would answer our prayers were finally behind us. To be faithful is certainly a wonderful thing. But, honestly, there's no denying the pure fear of losing your family, the same fabric as you, the people who identify who you are. It's a lonely feeling to think of your sister leaving you. As it happened Karol and I have lost Honey, our only other sister since Karol's ordeal in 2015. It was during the night on Sunday, November 24th, 2019, the angels came. In the early morning she was found already gone. There was no warning, no time to say goodbye. The loss is as gripping today for me as it was the moment, we got the call. Karol, my junior of nine- and one-half years has consoled and counseled me many times since then. When we were younger, she was the emotional one, but the brain injury has affected her emotional expression. This only means I'm the one falling apart, and Karol is the one lifting me up. She's so strong, so led by her faith.

Karol had been moved from Kindred in the Gables to Health South in Cutler, where she would remain until Christmas. She had a lot of hard work ahead, but Terry was by her side, and she was awake, thank God. I wasn't aware but Mary Ann pulled her phone out to video our reunion. But I was glad to be able to watch it, many times. We couldn't let go. This truly was one of the best moments in my life. Seeing Karol awake and talking, the relief and the joy is impossible to put into words. Over the next few days, we stayed with Karol as much as was allowed. I was glad Mary Ann asked all the questions and Terry explained everything. The only thing I could is hold on to my sister and look into her eyes, wide open, and her, smile, I had missed that so.

There's an addendum I feel should be included, a brief note about Sarah Frances. She was just preparing to return to Palm Beach for her second year of college. I hadn't planned on this talk and was a little unsure after I spoke if it was bad timing or too much pressure. I told Sarah I felt like her mom wouldn't want her to interrupt her education. There was no hesitation. Her mother's daughter, Sarah planned to continue, which she did. The faith in this family brought them through that time. Today, Sarah Frances, just recently married this past spring, finished her education through a master's program and has recently accepted a Social Services supervisory position for the low country of South Carolina providing care for at risk children. Her parents couldn't be prouder.

The devil is alive and well on this earth, with all the hatred happening.

CPSIA information can be obtained
at www.ICGtesting.com
Printed in the USA
LVHW030459281122
733996LV00004B/6